American College of Physicians
Home medical guide to epilepsy

DATE DUE			

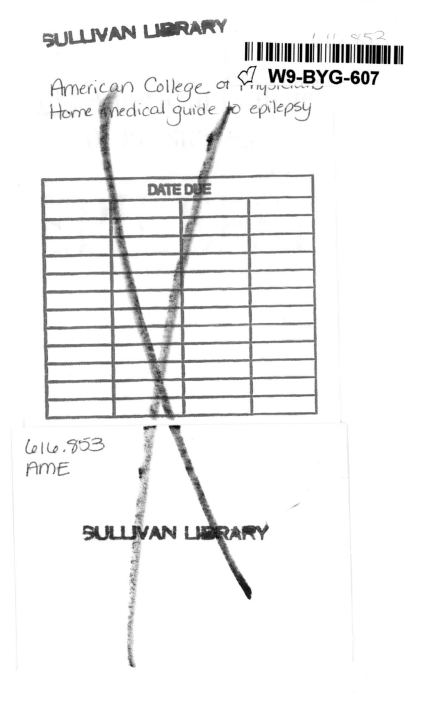

DK American College of Physicians

of Physicians

HOME MEDICAL GUIDE *to*

EPILEPSY

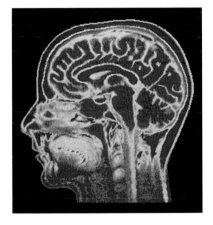

MEDICAL EDITOR
DAVID R. GOLDMANN, MD
ASSOCIATE MEDICAL EDITOR
DAVID A. HOROWITZ, MD

A DORLING KINDERSLEY BOOK

IMPORTANT

The American College of Physicians (ACP) Home Medical Guides provide general information on a wide range of health and medical topics. These books are not substitutes for medical diagnosis, and you should always consult your doctor on personal health matters before undertaking any program of therapy or treatment. Various medical organizations have different guidelines for diagnosis and treatment of the same conditions; the American College of Physicians–American Society of Internal Medicine (ACP–ASIM) has tried to present a reasonable consensus of these opinions.

Material in this book was reviewed by the ACP–ASIM for general medical accuracy and applicability in the United States; however, the information provided herein does not necessarily reflect the specific recommendations or opinions of the ACP–ASIM. The naming of any organization, product, or alternative therapy in these books is not an ACP–ASIM endorsement, and the omission of any such name does not indicate ACP–ASIM disapproval.

DORLING KINDERSLEY
LONDON, NEW YORK, AUCKLAND, DELHI,
JOHANNESBURG, MUNICH, PARIS, AND SYDNEY

DK www.dk.com

Senior Editors Jill Hamilton, Nicki Lampon
Senior Designer Jan English
DTP Design Jason Little
Editor Irene Pavitt
Medical Consultant Peter B. Crino, MD PhD

Senior Managing Editor Martyn Page
Senior Managing Art Editor Bryn Walls

Published in the United States in 2000 by
Dorling Kindersley Publishing, Inc.
95 Madison Ave., New York, New York 10016

2 4 6 8 10 9 7 5 3 1

Based on an original work by Dr. Matthew Walker and
Professor Simon D. Shovron.

Library of Congress Catalog Card Number 99-76862
ISBN 0-7894-4170-5

Reproduced by Colourscan, Singapore
Printed and bound in the United States by Quebecor World, Taunton, Massachusetts

Contents

Introduction

What do the following people have in common: Julius Caesar, the apostle St. Paul, Dostoyevsky, Vincent van Gogh, the prophet Muhammad, Joan of Arc, the Buddha, Edward Lear, Gustave Flaubert, and Alexander the Great? The answer is that they probably all had epilepsy.

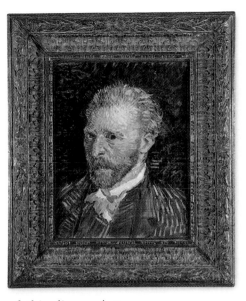

People from all walks of life suffer from epilepsy, and it is therefore somewhat surprising that any mis-understandings regarding the nature of this disease arise. In fact, many people hide their epilepsy from friends, employers, and sometimes even members of their own family because they worry about the possibility of stigma or prejudice.

Epilepsy has undoubtedly achieved an unenviable image in people's minds, perhaps largely because of its unpredictable, dramatic, and sometimes frightening effects. Although there are many different types of seizures, as will be explained later, it is the convulsion – falling to the ground, frothing at the mouth, flailing of the limbs – that comes to most people's minds when the word *epilepsy* is mentioned. It is this dramatic event

EPILEPSY AMONG THE FAMOUS
Vincent van Gogh, the 19th-century Dutch painter, is believed to have suffered from epilepsy.

7

that has always fueled people's imaginations; epileptic seizures are mentioned in the earliest Babylonian and Hebrew tracts. In ancient Greece, at a time when people were obsessed with gods and spirits, Hippocrates was one of the first people to try to dispel the superstition that surrounded epileptic seizures. He firmly believed that epilepsy originated in the brain and even went as far as condemning those who proposed that epilepsy was caused by demonic possession.

Yet for the next 2,000 years, this theory of demonic possession led to people with epilepsy being shunned, locked away, and subjected to unpleasant, painful, and humiliating ordeals in the name of a cure. The account of the death of the English king Charles II includes a description of the treatment of his seizure. This included bleeding him, giving him substances that caused him to vomit, administering repeated enemas, shaving his head, blistering his skin, and finally forcing an unpleasant concoction down the dying king's throat.

Even as recently as the 19th century, circumcision and castration were proposed as cures for epilepsy. It was not until the end of the 19th century that the first effective medication, potassium bromide, was introduced; since that time, drug treatment has allowed the majority of people with epilepsy to lead normal, seizure-free lives.

To a certain extent, however, a stigma is still attached to what is a common condition. Almost every one of us knows someone who has epilepsy, although we may be unaware that he or she is affected.

How Many People Suffer from Epilepsy

- 2.3 million Americans have been diagnosed with epilepsy.
- Seizures will develop in 180,000 Americans of all ages this year.
- 300,000 children aged 14 years and younger have been diagnosed with epilepsy.

══ HOW COMMON IS EPILEPSY? ══

Epilepsy is extremely common. Each year, about 150,000–200,000 people in the US develop epilepsy. The majority are either children or elderly people, although the condition may develop between the ages of 20 and 50.

The chance of an individual developing epilepsy is about 1 in 30. However, only one in 200 people, or approximately 2.3 million people in the US, has active epilepsy. This implies that most people who have epilepsy eventually get better, and indeed this is the case. In about six out of every ten people, the condition improves without treatment.

Epilepsy affects males and females almost equally, although certain types of epilepsy are more common in one sex or the other. It affects all classes and all races.

Thus epilepsy is extremely common and may get better. This is an important message for all those who develop the condition.

WHO GETS EPILEPSY?
In most people who have epilepsy, the condition begins in childhood or after the age of 50

KEY POINTS

- There are many types of epilepsy and seizures.
- Epilepsy usually begins in childhood or old age.

What are seizures and epilepsy?

Seizures take many forms. They all originate in the brain, but different types of seizures arise in different parts of the brain.

The brain is involved in the formation of our emotions, thoughts, and memories, in the control of our movements, and in the appreciation of sensations, sounds, smells, tastes, and sight.

It is divided into two halves joined in the middle; the right half controls the left-hand side of the body, and the left half controls the right-hand side. Each half (or hemisphere) is further divided into four lobes (see the box opposite). For most of us, the left half is "dominant," controlling how we form and understand language.

Damaging one part of the brain affects its ability to function. For example, damage to the left occipital lobe results in the inability to see anything on the right; damage to the right frontal lobe causes a person to be paralyzed on the left side. Conversely, activating the left

SWEET SENSATIONS
When we smell something, we are activating the temporal lobe of our brain. If this part of the brain becomes damaged, our sense of smell may become impaired.

The Structure of the Brain

This view of the left side of the brain shows the brain stem, the cerebellum, and one of the two cerebral hemispheres. Each hemisphere is composed of four lobes, and each lobe has specific functions.

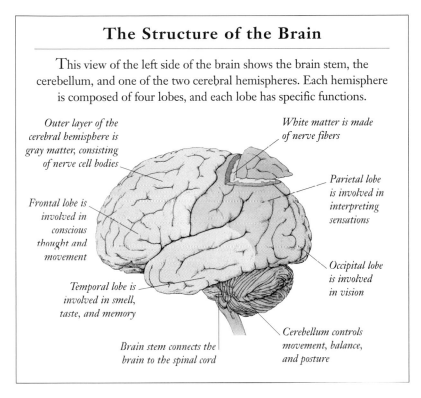

Outer layer of the cerebral hemisphere is gray matter, consisting of nerve cell bodies

White matter is made of nerve fibers

Frontal lobe is involved in conscious thought and movement

Parietal lobe is involved in interpreting sensations

Temporal lobe is involved in smell, taste, and memory

Occipital lobe is involved in vision

Brain stem connects the brain to the spinal cord

Cerebellum controls movement, balance, and posture

The Lobes of the Brain

Each of the four lobes of each cerebral hemisphere has its own particular physical and mental functions. These can be impaired by brain damage.

FRONTAL LOBE
Involved in the control of movement.

PARIETAL LOBE
Involved in the interpretation of sensations.

TEMPORAL LOBE
Involved in the appreciation of smells and tastes and the formation of memories.

OCCIPITAL LOBE
Involved in vision.

occipital lobe with an electric current, for example, results in the person seeing colored images or shapes on the right-hand side, and stimulation of the right frontal lobe causes the left part of the body to move.

A seizure can be likened to an electrical storm. This storm can be confined to one part of the brain, spread to other parts, or involve the whole brain at once. Seizures that start in one part of the brain are known as "partial seizures," and those that start in both halves at once are known as "generalized seizures." The symptoms experienced by the person or seen by others depend on where the seizure starts and how far and how quickly it spreads.

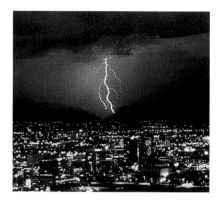

ELECTRICAL STORM
An epileptic seizure is like an electrical storm. It can be confined to one part of the brain, it may spread to other parts, or it may involve the whole brain.

In the next section, we define the different types of seizures in some detail.

TYPES OF SEIZURES

Almost all seizures are sudden, short-lived, and self-limiting. Most occur spontaneously without warning, and, as explained above, the form of the seizure depends on the part of the brain involved. Their classifications are listed in the table opposite.

PARTIAL SEIZURES

● **Simple partial seizures,** during which there is no loss of consciousness, are confined to one small part of the brain. They are often classified according to the lobe (temporal, frontal, parietal, or occipital) in which the seizure starts.

In temporal lobe seizures, the patient may experience a feeling of intense fear, vivid memory flashbacks, intense déjà vu (a feeling of having been in an identical situation before), and unpleasant intense smells or tastes. We can all experience some of these from time to time, and, of course, they are not usually seizures. For example, déjà vu is a common and normal experience. The main difference is that, in people with epilepsy, these things happen regularly and without reason, they are short-lived, and they occur with an intensity that is rare in everyday life.

In frontal lobe seizures, there may be uncontrolled jerking of one arm or leg or the head, and the eyes may turn to one side.

In parietal lobe seizures, the patient may experience tingling down one side of the body.

In occipital lobe seizures, the patient may experience flashing lights in one-half of the field of vision. The seizure usually lasts a matter of seconds.

- **Complex partial seizures** are the next stage up from simple partial seizures. The seizure involves a larger part of the brain and spreads to enough of the brain that the patient is no longer aware of his or her environment and is thus unconscious. The spread of the seizure can be either so fast that the patient does not experience the simple partial seizure, or so slow that the patient has, for example, a feeling of déjà vu, a strange unpleasant taste, or an awareness of colored flashing lights lasting

Classification of Seizures

The broad categories of partial and general seizures can be divided into more specific subtypes.

PARTIAL SEIZURES	**A** Simple partial seizures
	B Complex partial seizures
	C Secondary generalized seizures
GENERALIZED SEIZURES	**A** Absence seizures (petit mal)
	B Myoclonic seizures
	C Clonic seizures
	D Tonic seizures
	E Tonic-clonic seizures (grand mal)
	F Atonic seizures

from seconds to a few minutes before actually becoming unaware of his or her surroundings.

During the seizure, it is quite common for complex, strange, or inappropriate actions to occur. They are known as automatisms. For example, the patient may fumble with clothing or make chewing movements.

Occasionally, the actions of the patient during the seizure are coordinated and can even take the form of running, dancing, undressing, or speaking nonsense. These seizures usually last only a matter of minutes, but they are occasionally prolonged. When the seizure stops, the patient is completely unaware of what he or she has done.

BRAIN ACTIVITY
The orange traces of this colored EEG show the electrical activity in the brain during an epileptic seizure. During a seizure, a chaotic and unregulated electrical discharge passes through the brain, causing an abrupt increase in activity.

● **Secondary generalized seizures** result from the spread of the seizure throughout both halves of the brain; the spread can be slow enough for the patient to have a warning (the aura) or so rapid that the patient loses consciousness without an aura. This spread is called secondary generalization, and the seizure takes the form of a generalized tonic-clonic seizure. In this seizure, the patient often becomes stiff (called the tonic phase) and may let out a high-pitched cry. He or she then falls and may become blue. The arms and legs jerk rhythmically (called the clonic phase); grunting, foaming at the mouth, tongue-biting, or incontinence may occur.

The seizure usually lasts for a few minutes, and afterward the patient is often confused, may not know where he or she is, and will often sleep. The aftereffects, or "postictal" phase, last for minutes or hours.

This type of seizure, which used to be called a grand mal attack, is now known as a tonic-clonic seizure and is sometimes referred to as a convulsion.

GENERALIZED SEIZURES

These seizures begin in both halves of the brain at once; therefore, there is no warning, and consciousness is lost immediately. Often this seizure is a tonic-clonic seizure (see above), but it can be a clonic seizure with no stiff phase or a tonic seizure with no shaking stage in which the patient just falls like a board.

There is a rare type of seizure, known as an atonic seizure, in which the patient just slumps to the ground but recovers very quickly.

There are also two other categories of generalized seizure: absences and myoclonic jerks.

- **Absence seizures** used to be called petit mal attacks. They are short blank spells, usually affecting children, that last just a matter of seconds and may be confused by teachers or parents with poor attention or loss of concentration. Children affected by absence epilepsy can have hundreds of these in a day, and often neither the child nor observers are aware of most of them because they are so brief. They are associated with a particular brain wave pattern that is discussed in the next chapter.

ABSENCE SEIZURES
The child stares blankly, stops talking, and becomes unaware during an absence seizure. It usually lasts for only a few seconds.

- **Myoclonic seizures** are usually seen in patients with other seizure types. They consist of very brief jerks of one limb or the whole body. The patient may describe suddenly dropping a cup of coffee as her hand flings up or being thrown to the ground.

From these descriptions, you can see that there are many different types of seizures. You are probably already aware that there are also other conditions that can be mistaken for an epileptic seizure, and they will be discussed in the next chapter.

THE CAUSE OF SEIZURE

All brain activity depends on the passage of electrical signals. The brain consists of millions of cells called neurons, which have bodies and long arms with branches known as axons. Neurons communicate with one another through a combination of electrical and chemical signals. Electrical signals pass down the axons like a telephone signal along a telephone line. When the signal reaches the end of the axon, it causes the release of a chemical that communicates with a nearby neuron body by means of special receivers called receptors. These receptors "excite" this neuron body, and, if the excitation is sufficient, a further signal is sent (or "fired") down its axon.

If only excitation took place in the brain, then eventually all the neurons would be firing together, thereby causing an "electrical storm" such as that seen in a seizure. But some neurons release a chemical from their axons that inhibits the surrounding neurons, preventing them from firing. The brain functions properly when there is a balance between the excitation and the inhibition. If there is either too much excitation or too little inhibition in a part of the brain (an imbalance), a seizure results. Epileptic seizures are a symptom of an underlying brain disturbance in the same way that a stomachache is a symptom of an underlying gut disturbance, such as food poisoning, ulcers, or appendicitis.

In partial seizures, the local imbalance between excitation and inhibition can result from local damage to the brain. This damage may be caused by any of a variety of factors, including lack of oxygen at birth, meningitis, or head injuries, or by abnormal tissue, such as a brain tumor or a defect in brain development.

In some cases, the underlying reasons for the partial seizures are not known.

In generalized seizures, the chemical imbalance affects a wide area of the brain, which often does not show any obviously abnormal structures. The imbalance can be caused by drugs such as cocaine and amphetamines, alterations of the body chemistry, excessive alcohol, or inherited or unknown factors.

How Nerve Signals Are Transmitted

Electrical signals are carried along a nerve cell on its axon. For a signal to cross the synapse (gap) between two nerve cells, chemical neurotransmitters must pass from the synaptic knob to receptors on the next cell.

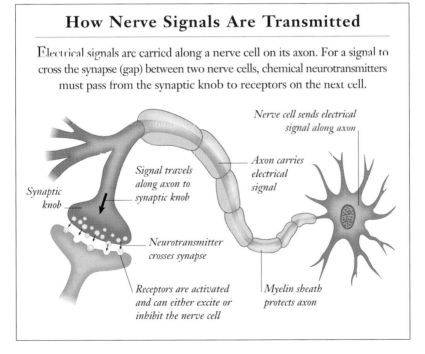

Nerve cell sends electrical signal along axon

Axon carries electrical signal

Signal travels along axon to synaptic knob

Synaptic knob

Neurotransmitter crosses synapse

Receptors are activated and can either excite or inhibit the nerve cell

Myelin sheath protects axon

EPILEPSY

Epilepsy is defined as a condition in which the person is prone to recurrent seizures. If you have one seizure brought on by excessive alcohol use and then you stop drinking, the chances of having another seizure are very small and a diagnosis of epilepsy is not justified. If, however, you have a number of seizures because part of your brain is damaged, the chances of having another seizure are very high and such a diagnosis is appropriate.

The decision about whether a patient does or does not have epilepsy is not always clear-cut. An individual's lifetime chance of having a seizure is about one in 30. We can considerably increase our chances of having a seizure by drinking excessively or taking certain drugs. However, most doctors diagnose patients as having epilepsy only if they have two seizures within a year because, in this instance, the chances of having a third seizure are probably over 80 percent, or 4 to 1.

ALCOHOL AND SEIZURES
Excessive alcohol, or withdrawal from alcohol, can cause seizures but not necessarily epilepsy.

The difficulty arises in patients who have had only one seizure. In this instance, the doctor usually assesses the chances of having another seizure, aided by various investigations and by knowledge of the type of seizure and the probable cause.

Most doctors usually do not prescribe drug treatment for a single seizure because of the low odds of having another one (less than 50/50) and the possible side effects of medication.

The second difficult question is, if a patient is diagnosed as having epilepsy, how many seizure-free years must pass before he or she is no longer considered to have epilepsy? Although there is no simple answer to this question, it is certainly true that many people with epilepsy eventually stop having seizures.

It is important to bear in mind that epilepsy is a range of symptoms, rather than a specific disease. A symptom is something that is experienced by patients and is indicative of an underlying disease. This is the case with epilepsy, which should be considered an indicator of some underlying brain problem. A wide spectrum of brain conditions can result in epilepsy.

WHAT IS AN EPILEPSY SYNDROME?

A syndrome is a medical term that refers to a specific condition in which characteristic groups of symptoms occur together. Syndromes are often named after the person who first described them.

For example, West syndrome is characterized by infantile spasms in which the baby suddenly bends over, by a particular brain wave pattern, and often by mental retardation in babies 3–12 months of age. Most of these children go on to have epilepsy that is difficult to treat and mental retardation. Thus a syndrome describes what happens but tells us nothing about the underlying cause of the seizures. There are, in fact, many causes of West syndrome.

The most common epilepsy syndromes are benign childhood epilepsy, with distinctive changes on the EEG, and primary generalized or generalized epilepsy. The table on page 20 outlines the features that characterize these two epilepsy syndromes.

Features of Epilepsy Syndromes

The two most commonly found types of epilepsy syndrome are benign childhood epilepsy and primary generalized epilepsy.

EPILEPSY SYNDROME	FEATURES
Benign childhood epilepsy with distinctive EEG changes	• Occurs between 2 and 14 years of age. • Can be inherited. • Seizures involve face, throat, and tongue, and consciousness is not lost. • Occasionally tonic-clonic seizures occur during sleep. • Typical EEG pattern. • Most get completely better, and drug treatment is usually not necessary.
Primary generalized epilepsy	• Usually occurs in childhood or adolescence. • Can be divided into many different syndromes. • Can be inherited. • Seizure types consist of a combination of absences, tonic-clonic seizures, and myoclonic seizures. • Seizures usually occur on or within a couple of hours of waking. • Typical EEG pattern. • Usually well controlled with medication.

KEY POINTS

- Seizures in different parts of the brain produce different effects.
- Seizures take many forms and can be compared to electrical storms in the brain.

Diagnosis of epilepsy

When a doctor first sees a patient whose symptoms suggest a possible diagnosis of epilepsy, there are two questions that need to be addressed. First, does the patient definitely have epileptic seizures, and, second, if the seizures are epileptic, what is the cause of the epilepsy?

IS IT EPILEPSY?

Many conditions can be confused with epileptic seizures. In adults, the most common are syncope (fainting), migraine, hyperventilation, panic attacks, and "pseudoseizures." In children, other conditions that can also commonly be confused with epilepsy include breath-holding attacks and night terrors.

FEELING FAINT
A person on the point of fainting may feel hot, dizzy, and nauseated. Sometimes a classic faint is confused with an epileptic seizure because both may cause jerking.

SYNCOPE

Syncope is the medical term for fainting, which occurs when not enough blood gets to the brain. The most common mechanism of syncope is the classic swoon (the vasovagal attack), in response to a strong unpleasant stimulus, such as seeing something disturbing, experiencing excruciating pain, or standing for a long period of time in a hot, enclosed space. Occasionally, syncope is due to an abnormal heart rhythm. It can also sometimes be precipitated by particular events, including coughing or urinating.

The classic vasovagal episode, or faint, is well known to everyone. The person feels dizzy, hot, and nauseated; becomes very pale; experiences graying of vision; and then slumps to the ground. At this point, blood flow to the brain increases, and the person comes around quickly. At first sight, it would seem difficult to confuse this with the seizures mentioned in the previous chapter. However, some jerking of the limbs can occur, especially if the person is propped up, because this position may prevent enough blood from reaching the brain. The jerking is occasionally prolonged but seldom has the coordinated pattern of a tonic-clonic seizure. In some partial seizures, the person may experience feelings similar to those of a faint; therefore, the two conditions are not always easy to distinguish.

MIGRAINE

As most people are aware, migraines often begin with a disturbance in vision or can be associated with tingling in the arm or face or, rarely, a disturbance of speech. It can be difficult to distinguish this from a simple partial seizure, especially because it is not uncommon to have a splitting headache after a seizure. However, consciousness is practically never lost with a migraine. There are also differences between the disturbances of vision in migraine and those experienced in epilepsy. Disturbances of vision in migraine usually evolve over minutes and have a simple form, such as circles of light or bright dots. Disturbances of vision in epilepsy evolve more rapidly, usually in just a few seconds, and are generally more complex, such as multicolored shapes or sometimes scenes or faces. In addition, if tingling occurs, it tends to spread slowly up the arm in migraine and rapidly in seizures. In most cases, there is little doubt about whether an attack is caused by migraine or epilepsy, but on some occasions it may present a diagnostic puzzle.

HYPERVENTILATION AND PANIC ATTACKS

Overbreathing, or hyperventilation, is not uncommon, especially in those under a lot of stress or in those who tend to panic (panic attacks). The feeling is usually described as a sudden difficulty in catching one's breath and a feeling of extreme emotional distress, although these symptoms do not always have to be present. During overbreathing, a person breathes out too much carbon dioxide, and when this happens the acidity of the blood changes. This in turn affects nerve activity and can cause tingling sensations in the fingertips and lips, spasms of the hand, lightheadedness, and even blackouts. These attacks are best treated with relaxation and breathing exercises. Breathing into a paper bag during an attack enables a person to take in the carbon dioxide that he is exhaling and thereby prevent or reverse the effects of hyperventilation.

CONTROLLING BREATHING
Breathing into a paper bag during hyperventilation will cause carbon dioxide to be reinhaled, restore the level of acidity in the blood, and thereby calm breathing.

"PSEUDOSEIZURES"

Pseudoseizures are often the most difficult to distinguish from true epileptic seizures. These attacks are "all in the mind," although they are usually involuntary and occur without conscious motivation. Occasionally these attacks are "put on," but for the most part the patient has little control, and they can be likened to an emotional out-burst. The patient may fall, appear to lose consciousness, and then thrash around or lie motionless. These attacks often have some deep-rooted emotional basis and may require psychiatric treatment. They do not respond to drugs for epilepsy. When it is difficult to distinguish these attacks from an epileptic seizure, patients may be admitted to the hospital for close observation.

BREATH-HOLDING ATTACKS

Toddlers can hold their breath until they turn blue and may resort to this if they do not get their own way. Usually the attack stops there, but occasionally a strong-willed toddler will hold the breath until he or she passes out. These attacks do not require drug treatment, and they usually stop of their own accord.

NIGHT TERRORS

Night terrors usually affect children under the age of five years. A few hours after falling asleep, the child appears to wake, is terrified, and cannot be comforted. In the morning, the child generally has no memory of the previous night's events. Although night terrors may concern the parents, they are completely innocuous and do not require treatment.

DIAGNOSING THE PROBLEM

The most important diagnostic tool is the medical history, the question-and-answer session that occurs between a patient and his or her doctor. To determine whether the episodes are seizures, the doctor asks for a detailed description of what happens. Obviously, since consciousness may be impaired during the seizure, it is important to have someone present who has seen an episode in order to help with the description. A video of the episode is even better.

The doctor will be interested in the underlying cause of the seizures and will ask questions about alcohol use, head injuries, problems with birth, and whether the patient has had meningitis or has a family history of epilepsy. He or she will also be interested in the impact that epilepsy has on the patient's life and will ask about the patient's job and home life. Finally, the doctor will examine the patient, looking for clues to any underlying brain abnormality, and check the heart, especially if syncope is suspected.

TESTING REFLEXES
Leg reflexes form part of the detailed neurological examination that your doctor will carry out to help him or her diagnose the cause of your seizures.

A detailed neurological examination involves checking the eyes, the face, coordination, power and sensation in the limbs, and the reflexes in the arms, legs, and feet. In addition to blood chemistry and various other routine tests, the doctor may request one or more special investigations to assist him or her in making a diagnosis: electroencephalography (EEG), and computerized tomography (CT) scanning or magnetic resonance imaging (MRI) of the head.

ELECTROENCEPHALOGRAPHY (EEG)

This is literally "recording the electricity from the brain." Wires are attached to different parts of the head and are then connected to an amplifier, which magnifies the small electrical signal from the brain and records this signal onto paper. An EEG tracing is a recording of the internal electrical patterns of the brain and does not involve the passage of any electricity into or out of the brain. It is thus a harmless and painless investigation that is of great use to the doctor.

Normally, the tracing shows a wave pattern (the "brain waves"), with one wave occurring about every tenth of a second. The waves slow down during sleep and speed up when the patient is alert. If the patient is prone to epilepsy, the electrical pattern may be different and can show spikes or spike/wave patterns. In about half of the people who have epilepsy, an EEG tracing can pick up spikes even when the person is not having a seizure. If spikes are present, there is a 99-percent chance that the person has epilepsy. EEG is occasionally performed while the patient is asleep because spikes are more likely to be picked up during this period.

A particular EEG pattern, called "3 per second spike and wave," is especially significant. It is seen in patients with absence epilepsy, which requires a specific form of drug treatment and has a good outcome.

EEG performed during a seizure, especially if the patient is videotaped at the same time, is of great use in the diagnosis of patients whose condition is unclear. The video recordings identify exactly where the seizure starts, which is necessary, for example, in assessing patients for epilepsy surgery. One such test is called video telemetry. This involves admitting the patient to the hospital for several days, during which time he or she is constantly monitored by EEG and video. Sometimes it is also necessary to reduce or withdraw the patient's anticonvulsant medication in order to induce a seizure while he or she is being monitored.

CT SCANNING

Computerized tomography, or CT, scanning is literally the use of a computer to give detailed pictures of "slices" of the brain, much like the slices through a loaf of bread. This diagnostic technique uses X-rays. However, unlike a conventional skull X-ray, in which X-rays are fired at one side of the head with a photographic plate on the other side, in a CT scan, X-rays are fired at different angles and picked up by "receivers." The information obtained during CT scanning is then analyzed by a computer that displays the X-ray signal as a series of pictures of slices through the patient's skull and brain.

By using this technique, it is now possible to discover brain abnormalities, such as tumors, strokes, hemorrhages, and atrophy – the last of these possibly indicating Alzheimer's disease. However, CT scanning is gradually being replaced by magnetic resonance imaging, or MRI (see opposite page), in the diagnosis of the causes of epilepsy, because MRI is a much more sensitive test and also gives much clearer pictures of brain structures.

During a CT scan, the patient has to lie with his or her head stationary in the scanner for a number of minutes. However, this is an entirely painless procedure.

Occasionally, a dye is injected into a vein in the arm to highlight certain parts of the brain in order to gain more information from the scan.

SEEING INSIDE THE BRAIN
CT scanning uses X-rays to create slice images of regions of the body. This colored scan shows a section of a normal brain.

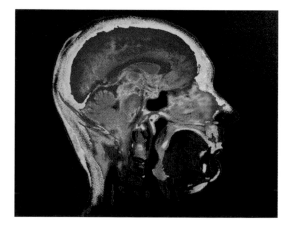

MAGNETIC RESONANCE IMAGING (MRI)

This procedure uses a large, powerful magnet, placed around the patient's head, instead of X-rays. The atoms in the brain orient themselves along this magnetic field. A burst of radio waves is then "fired" at the patient, and the hydrogen atoms in the brain wobble (resonate). As the hydrogen atoms gradually return to rest, they give off radio waves that are picked up by "receivers" and analyzed by a computer, result-

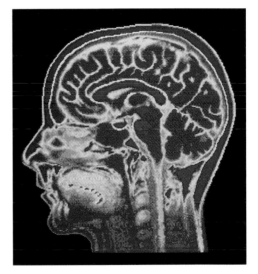

ing in detailed pictures of the brain. This technique is safe and entirely painless, but it does involve lying still in the enclosed space of a scanner for some time (usually 10–20 minutes), which some people find unpleasant. Also, as a result of the powerful magnets used, people with some types of metal implants, such as clips or wires from previous brain surgery or other operations and pacemakers, cannot be scanned.

MRI can detect many subtle and small abnormalities that were previously undetectable by CT scanning. As MRI techniques improve, the underlying cause of epilepsy can be discovered in more and more patients. MRI is especially useful in assessing the suitability of surgical treatment for patients who have not responded to drugs (see p.47). Computer analysis can also be used to calculate the relative size of different brain structures. This is important in, for example, analyzing certain areas of the brain (especially an area known as the hippocampus) that, when damaged, can cause seizures.

MRI BRAIN SCAN
This color-enhanced MRI scan shows a cross section of a normal brain. MRI is increasingly being used to detect brain abnormalities.

Causes of Epilepsy from Birth to Old Age

This chart lists the likely causes of epilepsy in both children and adults. Birth trauma and genetic disease may cause childhood epilepsy, while in adults brain tumors or strokes are common causes.

- Inherited brain diseases (e.g., tuberous sclerosis).
- Inherited epilepsies (e.g., primary generalized epilepsy).
- Birth trauma.
- Febrile convulsions.
- Brain infections (e.g., meningitis, encephalitis, brain abscesses).
- Alcohol and recreational drugs (e.g., cocaine, amphetamines, "Ecstasy").

- Head trauma.
- Blood chemical abnormalities (e.g., low calcium, magnesium, or glucose).
- Cerebral hemorrhages.
- Brain tumors (e.g., gliomas, meningiomas).
- Strokes.
- Dementia (e.g., Alzheimer's disease).

THE CAUSES OF EPILEPSY

As has been emphasized, epilepsy is a symptom and not a disease. There are many causes, such as infections, head injuries, brain tumors, brain injuries at birth, and inherited diseases (see above). Occasionally, epilepsy can appear many years after the damage has occurred. For example, it is not uncommon for people who have sustained a brain injury in childhood to have their first attack of epilepsy in their 20s.

For many sufferers (approximately 70 percent), no cause is ever found. Genetic factors are likely to play a role in the generalized forms of epilepsy, and some forms of epilepsy are hereditary, but in most cases this is not so. Except in a few genetically inherited conditions that can cause epilepsy, the risks of passing the condition on to your offspring are very small.

KEY POINTS

- Many conditions are confused with epilepsy, the most common being fainting, migraine, panic attacks, "pseudoseizures," and breath-holding attacks and night terrors in children.
- Epilepsy can be caused by infections, head injuries, brain tumors, brain injuries at birth, and inherited diseases, but often the cause is not known.
- Investigations for diagnosing epilepsy include EEG, CT scan, and MRI, but the patient's medical history is of greatest importance in making the diagnosis.
- Risks of passing epilepsy on to offspring are very small.

Treatment of epilepsy

Much can be done to prevent a person from being injured during an epileptic attack by following a few simple procedures. Drug therapy can help cut down the number of such attacks.

FIRST AID TREATMENT
Although a major seizure is frightening to watch, stay calm and loosen any tight clothing to make sure that the person can breathe.

MANAGING SEIZURES

Seizures are often frightening to watch, especially because the person may turn blue, have wild, jerking movements, foam at the mouth, and cry out. People often wish to intervene by placing an object in the person's mouth to keep him or her from "swallowing

What to Do During a Seizure

There are a few simple procedures that should be followed if you are present during a seizure. The most important thing is to stay calm and let the seizure run its course.

- During a seizure, the patient should be laid on the ground, away from objects that can cause injury. The head should be cushioned, and the patient should not be restrained in any way.
- After the seizure, the patient should be placed in the recovery position, and someone should remain with the patient until he or she is fully recovered.
- Sometimes, confusion can mimic aggression. In these cases the patient should not be restrained but gently coaxed out of danger. At this stage, if anything is blocking the airway, it should be cleared.
- If the seizure lasts longer than 5 minutes, or if the patient is having repeated seizures without regaining consciousness, call an ambulance.

the tongue" and by calling an ambulance. The former intervention can, however, be dangerous. Objects should not be placed in the patient's mouth during the seizure because the patient may bite the hand of the helper or the object, resulting in damage to the teeth and mouth.

If you are experiencing a lot of seizures, having someone call an ambulance every time is embarrassing and usually unnecessary as well.

The chart at the top of this page shows the correct procedure in the event of a seizure.

Some patients have recurrent prolonged seizures, and occasionally caregivers will be asked to give these patients a drug called diazepam, either by mouth or as

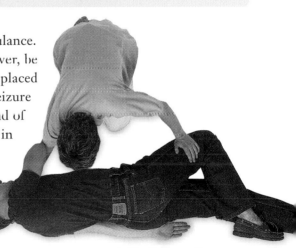

THE RECOVERY POSITION
To place someone in the recovery position, gently pull the person toward you with one hand on the lower part of the body. Protect the patient's face with the other hand.

a suppository, in order to stop the seizure. This policy should be discussed with the doctor in charge of the care of any patient who has repeated episodes of seizures lasting longer than 20–30 minutes, because immediate drug therapy may be beneficial to the patient and eliminate the need to go to the hospital.

LONG-TERM TREATMENT

The aim of long-term treatment is to stop all seizures, and this can be achieved in about 80 percent of all patients. The following are the three main ways in which to achieve this:

- Avoiding those things that cause seizures.
- Drug treatment.
- Brain surgery.

Very occasionally, patients who have warnings that last a long time before losing consciousness are able to control their seizure and prevent loss of consciousness. This is sometimes achieved by intense concentration during the warning period.

TRIGGER FACTORS
Very rarely, certain pieces of music can trigger an epileptic seizure in susceptible people.

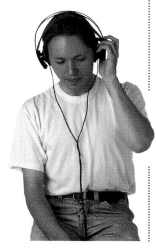

AVOIDING TRIGGERS

In many patients, avoiding certain factors will lessen the frequency of seizures, and in a few it will prevent them altogether. Very rarely, seizures can be brought on by hearing particular pieces of music, reading, taking hot showers, or seeing certain patterns. These are referred to as "reflex epilepsies." Most people, however, never notice a specific trigger. There are nevertheless four things that can induce or worsen seizures in many people – excessive alcohol, lack of sleep, stress, and fever. Finally, a few patients are sensitive to flashing lights, which is called photosensitivity (see p.36).

ALCOHOL AND SLEEP DEPRIVATION

Often patients who have primary generalized epilepsies are particularly susceptible to seizures following binges of alcohol or sleep deprivation, and these are almost certainly two factors that all people with epilepsy should try to avoid. Indeed, alcohol abuse or suddenly stopping a pattern of alcohol abuse can induce seizures in almost anyone, and seizures are thus a common common complication of alcoholism. For those whose seizures are exacerbated by sleep deprivation, getting tired, missing sleep, and, in some cases, shift work are inadvisable.

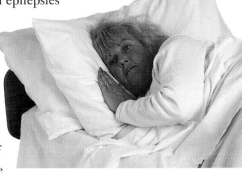

SLEEP DEPRIVATION
Many find that lack of sleep will prompt a seizure. People with epilepsy should make sure that they get regular and sufficient sleep.

STRESS

Although it is often difficult to identify the effects of stress, it can have a profound effect on seizure control. In addition, stress can affect whether patients take their medication (adherence) and thus indirectly worsen seizure control. Relaxation exercises and stress management can be beneficial. Often, counseling those who find it difficult to cope with epilepsy can help seizure control.

FEVER AND HIGH TEMPERATURES

Seizures can get worse during any illness, and this is especially so in young children if a fever is present. A high body temperature makes the brain more likely to have a seizure. Thus at the first signs of fever, the body temperature should be kept down with acetaminophen. Another instance in which the body temperature can rise, resulting in increased seizure frequency, is sunstroke, which is usually caused by a combination of excessive sun exposure and dehydration.

PHOTOSENSITIVITY

Recently, much has been made of light sensitivity (photosensitivity) and the relationship of seizures to video games, television, and computer screens. In fact, less than five percent of all people with epilepsy are sensitive to flashing lights. Photosensitivity seizures usually occur with lights that flicker from 5–30 times per second, and television and video games (both of which have flickering screens) can induce photosensitivity seizures in susceptible individuals. However, since children spend a large amount of time watching television and playing video games, any seizure that occurs while they are engaged in these activities may be purely coincidental.

Other common triggers include:
- Sunlight reflecting off water.
- Passing a line of trees through which the sun is shining.
- Stroboscopic lights (although there may be restrictions on the flash rate of strobe lighting, it is perhaps best avoided by susceptible individuals).

In some patients who have photosensitivity, avoiding triggers or taking certain precautions, such as wearing sunglasses in bright light, may be all that they need to do to prevent seizures.

The following precautions can be taken by those not on drug treatment to avoid television-induced seizures:
- Watch TV in a well-lit room.
- Watch the television from an angle.
- Sit at least 10 feet from the television set.
- Change channels with a remote control rather than getting too close to the screen.

Seizures are rarely triggered by films that are viewed in a movie theater, and computer screens usually operate at a high frequency in order to avoid provoking seizures.

However, in both of these instances, content, consisting of a changing geometric pattern at the correct frequency, can very occasionally provoke a seizure. Anticonvulsant drug treatment is generally effective in preventing photosensitivity seizures.

DRUG TREATMENT

Since the earliest times, people have been seeking effective drugs for epilepsy, and through the ages such cures as powdered human skull, vulture's blood, and mistletoe have all been tried without success. The first effective therapy, however, was reported in 1857 by Sir Charles Locock, an obstetrician who had an interest in epilepsy because of the mistaken idea, common at that time, that in some women epilepsy originated from their wombs. The drug he used was potassium bromide, and this remained the most effective therapy for epilepsy until 1912, when phenobarbital was introduced.

EARLY TREATMENT
Medication using the mistletoe plant was among the earliest attempts to treat people suffering from epilepsy.

The main drawbacks with bromides are their unacceptable side effects. In fact, the play-off of side effects against the effectiveness of an anticonvulsant drug is still at the heart of antiepileptic drug treatment.

HOW IS THE DRUG ABSORBED?

After it is swallowed, an anticonvulsant drug is absorbed into the bloodstream and then passes into the brain, where the drug acts. Whether an anticonvulsant is taken on an empty or a full stomach can affect the amount of drug that is absorbed. Consequently, the drug should generally be taken at the same time in relation to meals. Once the drug has circulated through the bloodstream, it is removed from the body. Depending on the specific drug, it is either broken down, or metabolized, by the liver or filtered out by the kidneys and passed in the urine. If a drug is removed from the body very quickly, it has to be taken frequently (3–4 times a day) to keep the blood levels of the drug reasonably high. Conversely, if a drug is removed from the body slowly, it can be taken only once a day.

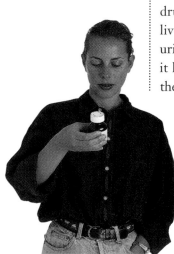

WHICH DRUG?
Your doctor will choose an anticonvulsant drug appropriate to your type of epilepsy and your needs.

HOW DO THESE DRUGS WORK?

It is not clear exactly how most anticonvulsant drugs work, but there do seem to be a number of important mechanisms. In an earlier chapter (see pp.16–17), it was explained that seizures may result when the excitation and inhibition that occur in the brain are not balanced. Some anticonvulsants correct this chemical imbalance. Others work by "stabilizing" neurons and thus preventing excessive firing.

THE RIGHT DRUG FOR THE PATIENT

Most anticonvulsant drugs are effective in the control of different types of epilepsy, and often it is just a matter of choosing the particular drug that suits the patient best. Interestingly, what may be a very effective drug in one patient may be useless in another one.

Some anticonvulsants, however, work only in certain forms of epilepsy. For example, ethosuximide is used just in order to treat absence epilepsy. Indeed, some anticonvulsants can even make certain types of epilepsy worse (for example, if carbamazepine is used to treat myoclonic seizures). A list of the drugs that are used most often in the treatment of particular seizure types is presented in the table on page 40.

SIDE EFFECTS

There are three main types of side effects of anti-convulsant drugs: dose-related side effects, individual or idiosyncratic side effects, and chronic side effects.

- **Dose-related side effects** are seen in all patients if the dose of the anticonvulsant drug is high enough. This is sometimes called drug intoxication. The amount of drug that can be tolerated varies from patient to patient. With most of the anticonvulsants, dizziness, double vision, unsteadiness, drowsiness, and headache are the most common dose-related side effects. They are alleviated by reducing the dose of the drug. In the case of drugs that are removed slowly from the body, it may take several days for the effects to be felt. Since many people become accustomed to some immediate side effects (especially drowsiness) after being on a drug for a little while, it is always prudent to give a drug a month or so before abandoning it because of mild side effects. Most of the anticonvulsants can also interfere with concentration and intellectual ability.

- **Idiosyncratic side effects** occur only in some people and are essentially allergies. They take the form of rashes or various blood disorders. Since these side effects do not depend on the size of the dose, the only way to overcome them is to discontinue the drug. If you develop a rash or other unusual symptoms, consult your doctor, who will modify your treatment.

- **Chronic side effects** occur after patients have taken a drug for many years. The chronic side effects of the newer anticonvulsant drugs thus are not as well documented as those of the older, more established drugs. The table on page 42 lists the more common side effects of some anticonvulsants.

Types of Seizures and Appropriate Drug Treatments

Some anticonvulsant drugs work for only particular forms of epilepsy, and it is important to choose the right drug to suit the patient and the type of seizures being experienced.

SEIZURE TYPE	DRUGS TRIED FIRST	OTHER DRUGS THAT ARE USED	
PARTIAL SEIZURES			
Simple partial	Carbamazepine	Felbamate	
Complex partial	Phenytoin	Gabapentin	
Secondary generalized	Valproate sodium	Lamotrigine	
		Phenobarbital	
		Primidone	
		Topiramate	
GENERALIZED SEIZURES			
Absences	Ethosuximide	Acetazolamide	Lamotrigine
	Valproate sodium	Clonazepam	
Atonic/Tonic	Valproate sodium	Acetazolamide	Lamotrigine
		Carbamazepine	Phenobarbital
		Clonazepam	Phenytoin
		Felbamate	Primidone
		Gabapentin	Topiramate
Tonic-clonic/Clonic	Carbamazepine	Acetazolamide	Phenobarbital
	Phenytoin	Felbamate	Primidone
	Valproate sodium	Lamotrigine	Topiramate
Myoclonic	Clonazepam	Acetazolamide	Primidone
	Valproate sodium	Phenobarbital	

DRUG INTERACTIONS

The levels of anticonvulsant drugs in the blood can be affected by other drugs, including other anticonvulsants, that interfere with the breakdown, excretion, and absorption of anticonvulsants. This results in either a fall in the blood level of the drug, causing seizures, or a rise in the blood level, causing side effects. It is thus important to check before taking any other medications, including those that can be bought without a prescription (see table on p.43 for a list of some of the commonly prescribed drugs that interact with anticonvulsants). When a new anticonvulsant is added to a patient's anticonvulsant drug treatment, it is often necessary to change the dose of the existing anticonvulsants and closely monitor blood levels.

Anticonvulsant drugs can also affect the blood levels of other prescription drugs. This effect is particularly important with oral contraceptives because many anticonvulsants increase the body's ability to break down contraceptives, rendering them ineffective. In this instance, higher contraceptive doses are required, or alternative methods of birth control may be recommended. Abnormal vaginal bleeding between the expected time of menses is a sign that the contraceptive dose may not be high enough and is not providing adequate protection. A similar increase in drug metabolism occurs when anticonvulsants are taken with warfarin, which stops blood from clotting, and this may result in the need for larger doses of warfarin.

ADJUSTING THE DOSE
Side effects, such as headache and dizziness, are a problem for some people and may mean that the dose needs adjusting.

STARTING AND STOPPING MEDICATION

Starting anticonvulsant drugs at a high dose can result in side effects. Anticonvulsants should therefore be

Possible Side Effects of Anticonvulsant Drugs

Anticonvulsants can produce three main types of side effect: dose-related, individual or idiosyncratic (rare allergic reactions), and chronic.

DOSE-RELATED	IDIOSYNCRATIC	CHRONIC
Double vision	Rash	Weight gain
Unsteadiness	Blood disorders	Vitamin deficiencies
Dizziness	Liver failure	Changes in facial
Sleepiness	Psychosis/depression	appearance
Headache		Acne
Stomach upset		Mood changes
Slowness		Sedation

introduced cautiously and the dose increased gradually. The final dose is determined by the balance between seizure control and side effects.

It is important to realize that individual patients require different doses because every patient metabolizes the drug at a different rate. Consequently, the final dose may be even greater than the generally recommended maximum dose for the drug. In this instance, there is usually no need for concern if the patient is not experiencing side effects. If a drug does not work or if the side effects are unacceptable, another drug is tried. Most patients can be controlled on a single type of anticonvulsant (known as monotherapy). For a smaller number of patients, two or more anticonvulsants are needed (known as polytherapy or combination therapy).

For the following reasons, the doctor will try, wherever possible, to avoid polytherapy:

● Some anticonvulsants interact with others.

- Side effects result more often from polytherapy than from monotherapy.
- It is difficult to remember to take many different drugs, and thus adherence is worse.
- There is a greater potential for mistakes.

When an anticonvulsant drug is being stopped, the dose must be decreased in gradual steps. A flurry of bad seizures can result from stopping an anticonvulsant suddenly, even if the drug had not seemed to be effective.

TAKING DRUGS REGULARLY

Taking a drug according to the doctor's instructions is known as adherence. Poor adherence – that is, failure to take a drug as instructed, whether by not taking the drug at all or by taking it irregularly – is a major cause of the failure of anticonvulsant drug treatment.

It usually takes several days or a few weeks for an anticonvulsant to be fully effective, and the occurrence of seizures is generally unpredictable. It is therefore imperative to take the drug regularly in order to prevent seizures. When patients are not having seizures, they feel perfectly well, apart from possible side effects of

Medications that Interact with Anticonvulsant Drugs

The commonly used drugs, both prescription and over-the-counter, that interact with anticonvulsant medication

MEDICATION	INDICATION
Allopurinol	Gout
Aminophylline	Chronic obstructive pulmonary disease (COPD)
Amiodarone	Heart rhythm disturbances
Antacids	Indigestion
Aspirin	Pain relief, stroke and heart attack prevention
Cimetidine	Indigestion, peptic ulcers
Diltiazem	Hypertension
Erythromycin	Infections
Fluoxetine	Depression
Folic acid	Vitamin deficiencies
Imipramine	Depression
Omeprazole	Indigestion, peptic ulcers
Verapamil	Hypertension

the anticonvulsants. Consequently, it is not surprising that most patients may miss an occasional dose, whether intentionally or inadvertently.

FOLLOWING A REGULAR ROUTINE

It is also very easy for patients on regular medication to forget whether they took the last dose. It is important to maintain a regular routine of taking the drug. Adherence is more difficult if a drug has to be taken more than twice a day, especially by children who do not want to take drugs at school. The situation becomes even worse if the patient is on polytherapy. A drug organizer, in which pills can be placed into compartments labeled by time and day, is often very useful. The patient need replenish the compartments only each week. Drug organizers are also useful for those who have poor memories or very busy routines.

STOPPING SUDDENLY

Occasionally patients decide to stop taking their drugs suddenly, often because of depression. This is potentially dangerous because it can lead to prolonged and frequent seizures. A similar effect may occur during periods of vomiting or diarrhea, when the anticonvulsant may not be absorbed. In these cases, it should be taken again or antivomiting (antiemetic) drugs should be prescribed by the doctor. Admission to the hospital may be necessary.

TAKING THE RIGHT DOSE

Finally, misunderstandings between doctors and patients can lead to mistakes in dosages. After a consultation, it is important to be clear about precisely how much of each drug must be taken. If necessary, the doctor should write down this information. When they are going to appointments, it is usually a good idea for patients to bring their drug or drugs with them. Answers to vague inquiries about drugs are rarely helpful.

MONITORING THE DRUGS

It is important to monitor the effectiveness of an anticonvulsant drug, and the best method is by noting seizure frequency. It is often surprisingly difficult to remember exactly how many seizures have occurred, and a written record is mandatory for patients who have frequent seizures. This seizure diary can be reviewed at each appointment with the doctor. It is imperative that patients learn to differentiate between their different types of seizures and to record the frequency of each of them separately. Information about when anticonvulsants were started should also be included.

The most important guide to dosage is how well the seizures are controlled and how a patient feels. However, occasionally it is helpful to take a blood sample (usually before the morning dose, if possible) to check the blood level of an anticonvulsant. Much is made of blood levels, but it is important to keep them in context. The levels at which most patients have good seizure control and few side effects give rise to the so-called therapeutic range of blood levels for some anticonvulsants. The problem is that we are all individuals, and an effective blood level for most people may be too high or too low for some people. Blood levels can, however, give the doctor a rough idea of whether the dose of a drug is adequate.

There are also other circumstances in which blood levels are very useful:

KEEPING A RECORD
Keep a record of all seizures and, if relevant, the obvious triggers. This record will help your doctor determine the effectiveness of your anticonvulsant medication.

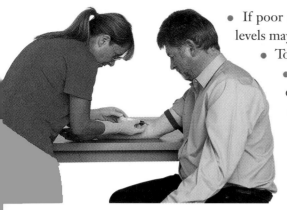

BLOOD LEVELS
A simple blood test is used to measure the levels of anticonvulsant medication in your blood. This can help your doctor determine whether the dosage of the drug is correct.

- If poor seizure control occurs because blood levels may have fallen.
  - To check for adherence to therapy.
    - If other drugs, including other anticonvulsants, that can interfere with the anticonvulsant therapy are started.
      - During pregnancy and illness, when blood levels of the drug (or drugs) may change.
      - In patients with severe learning difficulties, who may not be able to communicate whether or not they are experiencing side effects.

The various medications that are available for the treatment of epilepsy are described individually in the following chapter.

SURGERY FOR EPILEPSY

It has been estimated that as many as 600,000 patients with epilepsy in the US could benefit from epilepsy surgery. The potential for using surgery and its success rate may increase as the visualizing technique called magnetic resonance imaging (MRI) (see p.29) improves and the cause of seizures can be identified in more and more patients.

Epilepsy surgery is a major undertaking because it involves removing the part of the brain where the seizures originate. Obviously, this procedure is not without risk. Consequently, epilepsy surgery is reserved for those patients whose seizures are resistant to drug treatment (also known as drug-resistant, refractory, or pharmacoresistant patients) and in whom there is little chance of the seizures becoming less frequent.

CRITERIA

Before a patient is considered for epilepsy surgery, several criteria must be fulfilled:

• Seizures are one of the main causes of a patient's disability. A severely handicapped patient may have uncontrolled seizures that are only a minor problem compared with the rest of his or her disability problems.

• Both the doctor and the patient must agree that stopping the seizures would result in a significant improvement in the quality of life. For instance, undertaking brain surgery in someone who is suicidal or severely depressed for reasons other than epilepsy or in whom the epilepsy is of only small consequence is not recommended.

• The patient must be able to understand the possible risks and benefits of the epilepsy surgery.

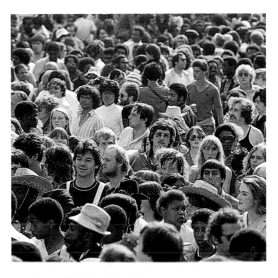

MANY COULD BENEFIT
Thousands of epilepsy sufferers could be helped by surgery, and it is likely to be more widely used as techniques are developed to identify the exact cause of seizures.

TESTS BEFORE SURGERY

Several tests have to be performed before the decision to opt for surgery is made:

• **Brain imaging** by MRI is used to identify any brain abnormalities that may be the cause of the epilepsy. If no such abnormality can be detected, this does not preclude epilepsy surgery but makes it less likely to be successful.

• **Psychological testing** is performed in order to identify whether any psychological problem or condition present is related to the part of the brain causing the seizures, to determine the importance of this part of the brain to a patient's memory and speech, and to provide a baseline for comparison after surgery has taken place. This usually involves administering a number of word, memory, and drawing and constructing tests that elucidate the function of different parts of the brain.

- **The measurement of the brain waves** by EEG also plays a pivotal role. Usually this involves a technique in which the brain waves are correlated with a video of the seizure to identify where the seizure starts. This is necessary to check that the abnormality seen on an MRI scan correlates with the part of the brain producing the seizures.

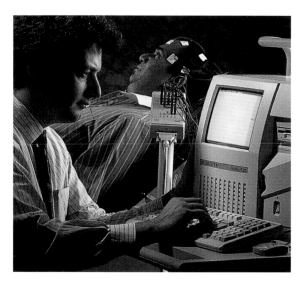

MONITORING THE BRAIN
By attaching small electrodes to the patient's scalp, a doctor can use an EEG machine to monitor brain activity. The patient's brain waves are displayed on the screen.

- **A sodium amytal test** is carried out in some cases. This test involves injecting the anesthetic agent sodium amytal into each side of the brain in turn. The drug is injected through a tube inserted into the main blood vessel in the groin and then passes up into the blood vessels that supply the brain.

Although this procedure sounds quite unpleasant, it is relatively painless and safe. As a result of the injection, each half of the brain is put to sleep in turn for a few minutes. During this period, the patient's memory and ability to name various objects are tested. Failure to complete the tests accurately indicates that the hemisphere of the brain put to sleep controls language and memory.

In most people, language is controlled by the left half of the brain and memory by both halves, but in a small number of people this pattern is lost. It is important to determine if this is the case because the effects of brain surgery on speech, understanding, and memory are vital factors in deciding whether surgery is indicated and what type of operation is possible.

• **Psychiatric assessment** is carried out in order to confirm that there is no mental illness, such as very severe depression or suicidal tendencies, that would prevent the patient from having brain surgery. If a mental illness is discovered, it must be successfully treated before surgery can be performed.

When all of the information is available, the patient's doctors meet with a brain surgeon in order to discuss the risks and benefits of epilepsy surgery for the patient.

Once these risks have been determined by the team of doctors, the risks and likely benefits are discussed with the patient, who then makes a decision.

PSYCHIATRIC ASSESSMENT
Many patients will be required to visit a psychiatrist before surgery in order to rule out any underlying mental illness.

THE OUTCOME

The outcome of epilepsy surgery depends largely on the type of operation, the part of the brain involved, and the underlying cause of the epilepsy.

For patients who have an identifiable defect in the temporal lobe of the brain, which is the most common situation, approximately 70 percent of them will become

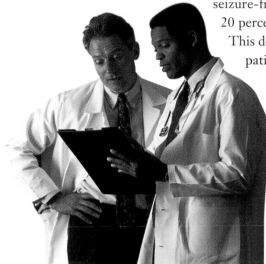

seizure-free after surgery, and another 20 percent will have some improvement. This does, however, still leave one in 10 patients who has no improvement or whose condition may even be worse after the operation than it had been before. Nevertheless, with advanced imaging and newer surgical techniques, the outcome of epilepsy surgery will continue to improve.

REACHING A CONCLUSION
Once all the tests have been completed, the risks and benefits of surgery for the patient are discussed by the doctor and surgeon.

KEY POINTS

- The aim of long-term treatment of epilepsy is to stop seizures.
- An anticonvulsant drug is chosen to suit the patient.
- Side effects of drugs can be dose-related, can occur in only some individuals, or can occur only in the long term.
- Some patients with epilepsy benefit from brain surgery.

Drugs used in the treatment of epilepsy

Most people who experience epileptic seizures find that their symptoms can be controlled with anticonvulsant drug therapy. Some of these drugs have been around for many years; others were developed much more recently.

ESTABLISHED DRUGS

Some of the most commonly used anticonvulsants, such as phenobarbital, have been in use since the early part of the twentieth century.

CARBAMAZEPINE

Carbamazepine has been around since the 1950s and has been found to be both safe and effective in the treatment of partial epilepsy and tonic-clonic seizures. It can, however, worsen absence seizures and myoclonic jerks. Occasionally, a rash or an abnormality of blood count can occur that requires the drug to be stopped. Too high a dose can lead to double vision, nausea, headache, and drowsiness. Carbamazepine is also available as a slow-release preparation that can be taken less frequently and has fewer side effects.

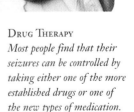

DRUG THERAPY
Most people find that their seizures can be controlled by taking either one of the more established drugs or one of the new types of medication.

51

CLONAZEPAM

Clonazepam is one of a group of drugs called benzodiazepines, which are better known for their use to treat anxiety and as sleeping pills. It is effective in absence seizures and other forms of epilepsy. In some patients, however, the drug ceases to be effective after a period of time, usually about three months. This phenomenon is called tolerance. As with all benzodiazepines, drowsiness and behavioral changes, especially aggression in children, are the main side effects.

ETHOSUXIMIDE

Ethosuximide is useful for only absence epilepsy; it is ineffective for other types of seizures. Some patients develop a rash, and side effects can include stomachache, fatigue, headache, and dizziness.

PHENOBARBITAL

Phenobarbital is one of the oldest established anticonvulsants and has been used since 1912. It is inexpensive and effective for most types of epilepsy but in recent years has gone out of favor because of its side effects. Originally, phenobarbital was used as a sleeping pill. It is therefore not surprising that some people become drowsy, although this drowsiness is mild and usually improves with time. Paradoxically, it can have the opposite effect in children, making them hyperactive and aggressive. In a few, phenobarbital can cause a rash and blistering. Too high a dose leads to drowsiness, impotence, depression, and poor memory. With long-term use, phenobarbital can coarsen facial features and decrease the body's stores of certain vitamins, such as folic acid and vitamin D.

PHENYTOIN

Phenytoin has been in common use since 1938. It was initially regarded as a breakthrough because it was as effective as phenobarbital but caused less drowsiness. Phenytoin is effective for partial seizures and tonic-clonic seizures. Some patients get a rash, in which case the drug must be stopped. Too high a dose can result in dizziness, increased seizures, drowsiness, unsteadiness, and double vision. Long-term use can result in swelling of the gums, coarsening of facial features, acne, growth of facial hair, and a decrease in the body's stores of certain vitamins, such as folic acid and vitamin D. Because of these potential long-term side effects, young people usually resist taking phenytoin.

PRIMIDONE

Primidone is broken down in the body to phenobarbital and, therefore, has the same side effects and uses as phenobarbital.

VALPROATE SODIUM

In France in the 1960s, valproate sodium was discovered by chance to be useful for the treatment of epilepsy. It is now the drug of choice for myoclonic seizures, light-sensitive epilepsy, and absence seizures. It is, however, effective for all types of epilepsy. It must be used cautiously in children under three, in whom it can occasionally cause severe liver damage. Some people experience a drop in the number of blood platelets, which are necessary for clotting.

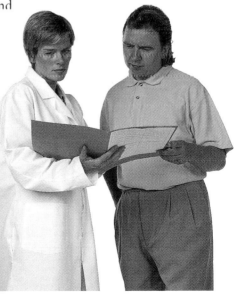

WEIGHT GAIN
Some patients find that they put on weight when taking medications such as gabapentin or valproate.

53

The most common side effects, however, are stomach upset, hair loss, tremor, swelling of the ankles, weight gain, and drowsiness, especially if given with phenobarbital. Valproate sodium is available as a slow-release preparation.

NEWER DRUGS

When anticonvulsant drugs are first developed, they are tried on patients with uncontrolled epilepsy (usually partial epilepsy) as an adjunctive therapy to existing anticonvulsant drug courses. If the drugs prove to be successful, they are approved for only this purpose. Some new anticonvulsants are, however, effective for other types of epilepsy. Doctors are permitted to prescribe drugs for such conditions, but they usually discuss this with the patient first.

GABAPENTIN

At present, gabapentin is licensed to be used only for partial epilepsy in combination with other anticonvulsants. It has few side effects, but at higher doses can cause dizziness, tremor, and drowsiness. Frequency of seizures can also increase in some patients. The drug can result in weight gain.

FELBAMATE

Felbamate is used alone or as adjunctive therapy for the treatment of partial and generalized seizures in adults. In children, it has been effective in the treatment of the Lennox-Gastaut syndrome, which is characterized by multiple seizure subtypes including atonic, tonic, and generalized seizures. The widespread use of felbamate was curtailed when cases of aplastic anemia and hepatic failure were documented in the US. Because of the

Anticonvulsant Drugs and their Year of FDA Approval

Some of the drugs used to treat epileptic seizures have been around for fifty years or more; others are fairly new.

DRUG (BRAND NAMES)	YEAR OF FDA APPROVAL
Phenobarbital (Barbita, Luminal, Solfoton)	1912
Phenytoin (Dilantin)	1953
Primidone (Mysoline)	1954
Ethosuximide (Zarontin)	1960
Carbamazepine (Tegretol)	1968
Diazepam (Valium)	1973
Clonazepam (Klonopin)	1975
Valproic acid (Depakene)	1978
Slow-release carbamazepine (Carbatrol, Tegretol XR)	1989
Gabapentin (Neurontin)	1993
Felbamate (Felbatol)	1993
Lamotrigine (Lamictal)	1994
Fosphenytoin sodium (Cerebyx)	1996
Topiramate (Topamax)	1996
Valproate sodium (Depacon)	1997
Tiagabine hydrochloride (Gabitril)	1997

risk of aplastic anemia, felbamate should be reserved for those patients in whom other therapies are not effective. Blood levels and liver function studies should be followed by an neurologist experienced in the use of felbamate. Common side effects include insomnia, anorexia, weight loss, dizziness, tremor, and lethargy.

LAMOTRIGINE

Lamotrigine originally had the same restricted use as gabapentin, but it is now licensed to be used as treatment for a variety of seizures and can be prescribed as monotherapy. It is potentially useful for most types of epilepsy. In a few patients, it causes a rash, which seems to be more likely to occur if a patient is started at too high a dose. Drowsiness, double vision, and dizziness may also result if the dose is too high.

TOPIRAMATE

Topiramate is a recently developed anticonvulsant used as an adjunctive treatment for a variety of seizure types. Side effects usually occur on starting treatment and include fatigue, stomach upset, unsteadiness, weight loss, and, rarely, kidney stones.

TIAGABINE HYDROCHLORIDE

Tiagabine hydrochloride was recently approved in the US as an adjunctive treatment for partial epilepsy. The main side effects experienced with this drug are dizziness, tremor, fatigue, depression, and, in some cases, diarrhea.

OTHER DRUGS

Drugs that have been developed primarily for the treatment of other conditions, such as diuretic drugs and drugs to treat anxiety and depression, have in some instances turned out to be valuable in the treatment of epileptic seizures as well.

ACETAZOLAMIDE

Acetazolamide is a diuretic (a drug that increases urination) and is mainly used to treat the eye condition glaucoma. It is, however, occasionally used as additional medication for patients with epilepsy.

The main problem with acetazolamide is that, after a few months, some patients develop a tolerance to the drug (i.e., the drug loses its ability to work effectively); it can also cause a rash. The other common side effects are excessive thirst, tingling in the hands and feet, fatigue, and loss of appetite.

DIAZEPAM

Diazepam is a benzodiazepine and is not generally used as regular medication but is effective in stopping a long seizure. For this purpose, it can be given by mouth or by suppository by caregivers or family members. In the hospital, it can be administered by intravenous infusion directly into a vein to stop prolonged seizures.

VITAMINS AND DIET

There is little evidence that either vitamins or diet help control seizures. Vitamin supplements may be necessary for those on long-term anticonvulsant treatment because some anticonvulsants can interfere with the body's vitamin stores (see pp.52–53).

A high-fat, low-carbohydrate diet called a ketogenic diet may help control seizures in some children with severe epilepsy and mental retardation. Unfortunately, this diet is unpleasant and difficult to maintain, so it is rarely used as a first-line therapy.

DRUGS FOR THE FUTURE

There are many studies of potential anticonvulsants taking place throughout the world. At this time, at least 10 new compounds look very promising. However, no drug so far has proved to be a cure-all, and it is still unclear why only some patients respond to only some drugs. Nevertheless, each new drug enables a greater number of patients to experience significant improvement in their epilepsy. It is hoped that, with a greater selection of drugs, fewer people will have uncontrolled seizures.

The newer drugs may have fewer side effects than the older drugs, but it is important to realize that long-term side effects of new drugs may be as yet unrecognized in contrast to those of older drugs, some of which have been used for over 50 years.

KEY POINTS

- Anticonvulsant medication will help control seizures in most people.
- Some of the drugs have been in use for more than 50 years.

Special situations

Febrile convulsions (experienced by young children) and status epilepticus seizure (a seizure that lasts more than 30 minutes) have particular characteristics that require special treatment.

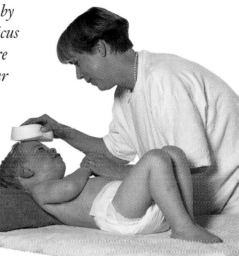

FEBRILE CONVULSIONS

This term is usually reserved for convulsions that occur in young children (three months to five years) when they have a fever ("febrile"). Febrile convulsions are important because they are common and often frightening to the parent. The condition should not, however, be referred to as epilepsy because it almost always disappears as the child grows older.

It is sometimes necessary to exclude brain infections such as meningitis as a cause. Occasionally, a lumbar puncture, in which a needle is inserted into the spine to withdraw some of the fluid that surrounds the brain, is needed to make sure that there is no brain infection. In most cases, there is no meningitis or other serious cause.

Indeed, over three percent of children between the ages of three months and five years will have at least one seizure associated with fever without underlying brain disease. It is more common in those with a relative who has had similar seizures or who has epilepsy.

CONVULSIONS IN CHILDREN
A high fever may cause a febrile convulsion in a young child. It is important to try to reduce a high fever with medication and by sponging with lukewarm water.

One-third of the children who have a febrile convulsion have subsequent febrile convulsions, but a very small number (less than five percent) develop true epilepsy.

If a child has had a convulsion with fever in the past, the child's temperature should be kept down during future febrile episodes with acetaminophen and by either sponging with lukewarm water or a lukewarm bath. In very susceptible children, diazepam suppositories can be given at the time of a fever to prevent a convulsion, and rarely a child may need regular anticonvulsant medication, usually valproate sodium or phenobarbital.

How a Lumbar Puncture Is Performed

A needle is inserted into the base of the spine to obtain a sample of cerebrospinal fluid. Examination of the cerebrospinal fluid can help in the diagnosis of such diseases as meningitis.

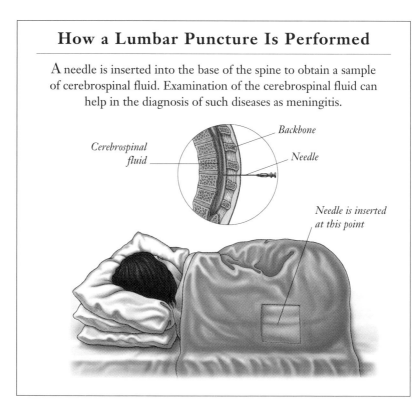

Cerebrospinal fluid

Backbone

Needle

Needle is inserted at this point

STATUS EPILEPTICUS

Most seizures last for only a few minutes. Some, however, can go on for longer – sometimes hours or even days. This is referred to as status epilepticus, defined as a seizure or a series of seizures that continues for more than 30 minutes, during which the patient does not regain consciousness. Any type of seizure may possibly lead to status epilepticus, but tonic-clonic status epilepticus (usually called convulsive status epilepticus) is a medical emergency.

As many as 10 percent of the patients with convulsive status epilepticus die. This is usually not as a result of the epilepsy itself but of the serious underlying cause of the status epilepticus (e.g., meningitis, stroke, or malignant brain tumors). About half the patients with status epilepticus have had chronic epilepsy, and, in these cases, sudden withdrawal of the anticonvulsant is one of the most common identifiable causes. About half of the patients have convulsive status epilepticus as their first seizure. When it occurs, urgent hospitalization and intravenous anticonvulsant therapy are required.

Many patients have an increasing number of seizures throughout the day leading up to convulsive status epilepticus, and in some – certainly those in whom status epilepticus occurs regularly – diazepam given by mouth or suppository will prevent the occurrence of the status epilepticus. Such a contingency plan needs to be made between the doctor and the caregivers or the family of the patient.

The other, nonconvulsive types of status epilepticus are not as serious. Often the patient will have just a prolonged typical seizure or series of seizures, leading to confusion that can go on for days. Nonconvulsive status epilepticus usually responds well to medication, such as diazepam administered by mouth.

PREGNANCY AND EPILEPSY

Careful monitoring of drug levels and frequency of seizures is necessary during pregnancy to ensure the health and well-being of both mother and baby.

CONCEPTION

Patients with epilepsy have lower birth rates. This is primarily due to social pressures, although epilepsy and its treatment can occasionally affect fertility. Furthermore, some anticonvulsants may decrease the patient's sexual drive.

The effectiveness of oral contraceptives can be reduced by anticonvulsants, and higher doses of the contraceptive may be necessary in order to provide adequate contraception. Bleeding between menstrual periods is a sign that the contraceptive is not working.

PREGNANCY

During pregnancy, about 30 percent of patients experience an increase in seizures, 20 percent experience a decrease in seizures, and 50 percent experience no change. The way the body deals with anticonvulsants changes during pregnancy, and regular monitoring of drug levels and seizures is required. Quite often, the dose of anticonvulsants has to be adjusted at some point during pregnancy. A woman may be tempted to reduce her medication during pregnancy because of a concern about the effects of the anticonvulsants on the developing child. Major convulsive seizures can, however, damage the developing child or result in miscarriage.

Consequently, the importance of good adherence cannot be overemphasized.

The risks of anticonvulsants to the development of the baby in the womb are small. The risk is higher in infants born to women on polytherapy and on high doses of anticonvulsants. The overall frequency of abnormalities of the baby at birth is about two percent for the general population, six percent for babies born to mothers on one anticonvulsant, and up to 20 percent for babies born to mothers on three different anticonvulsants. Therefore, before getting pregnant, the patient should be taking only the minimal amount of medication for adequate control of the epilepsy.

The most common significant abnormality in infants who are born to women with epilepsy is cleft lip or palate, which accounts for about one-third of the abnormalities that are seen. Spina bifida, a more serious consequence of anticonvulsant drug treatment, is most common when the mother is taking valproate sodium (1–2 percent of births) or carbamazepine (0.5–1 percent of births). Patients on these medications can have ultrasound and blood tests during pregnancy to detect spina bifida early enough for the pregnancy to be safely terminated if the parents desire. All women who are on anticonvulsant therapy should be given folic acid pills before conception and throughout the first three months of pregnancy. This naturally occurring vitamin reduces the risk of miscarriage and fetal malformation, particularly spina bifida. Therefore, there is a good argument for all women to take folic acid during these periods regardless of whether they have epilepsy or not.

CLOSE MONITORING
Medication must be carefully monitored during pregnancy to make sure that no harm comes to either the mother or the unborn baby.

63

During the last month of her pregnancy, vitamin K supplements should be given to the mother. The newborn child should also receive vitamin K supplements because anticonvulsants decrease the amount of this vitamin in the body. If the newborn child does not have enough vitamin K, his or her blood may not clot properly, and problems with bleeding and brain hemorrhage may result.

BREAST-FEEDING

Women with epilepsy who are taking anticonvulsants can usually breast-feed safely because very little of the medication is passed into the breast milk. The exceptions are high doses of either ethosuximide or phenobarbital, which are excreted in breast milk in significant quantities. Phenobarbital in breast milk can make the baby drowsy.

KEY POINTS

- Convulsions that occur in young children only at the time of a fever usually do not lead to epilepsy.
- Seizures that last for hours or days are known as status epilepticus. Convulsive status epilepticus is a medical emergency.
- During pregnancy, the risks of anticonvulsants to the baby are small and certainly smaller than the risks of the mother having uncontrolled convulsions.
- It is generally safe for women to breast-feed while taking anticonvulsants.

The social implications

Although we have spent a large part of this book dealing with the medical aspects of epilepsy, it is important to realize that there are many social implications of epilepsy, particularly with regard to driving, employment, schooling, and relationships.

SAFE DRIVING
A person with epilepsy can drive only when he or she has been symptom-free for a specific period of time, as determined by each state.

Unfortunately, society still places extra pressures on those who have epilepsy, although sometimes with justification, as in the case of driving.

DRIVING

Seizures experienced while driving are still one of the most common preventable causes of traffic accidents. The rules about driving vary from state to state, but a number of requirements are common to the majority of states. The following discussion is an over-view of state regulations. For specifics, contact your state motor vehicle department.

Most states require that people with epilepsy be seizure-free for a specified period of time and that they

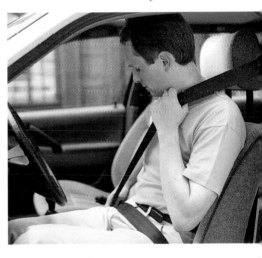

Criteria for Driving

A driver's license can be considered by the state motor vehicle department when the criteria below are fulfilled:

- No epileptic seizures have occurred for a certain period of time, specified by the state.
- A doctor determines an applicant's ability to drive safely, and updated medical reports are submitted to the state agency.

submit a doctor's determination of their ability to drive safely and periodic medical reports to the department of motor vehicles.

In those states that stipulate a seizure-free period, usually one year, a license may be issued or renewed after a shorter time under certain conditions. These exceptions include an isolated seizure if further seizures are considered unlikely by the person's doctor, an isolated seizure resulting from a missed dose or a change in medication ordered by the doctor, a pattern of seizures occurring only during sleep, and a pattern of a long aura preceding a seizure.

Many states issue licenses with restrictions that may be removed once a driver with epilepsy meets the regular licensing requirements. The restrictions include driving only during the day, only for a certain distance, or only in an emergency.

When applying for or renewing a driver's license, people with epilepsy must report the condition. After being licensed, they must give the state agency medical updates. Some states require reports for only a specified period of time, while others require them for as long as a driver is licensed. Six states – California, Delaware, Nevada, New Jersey, Oregon, and Pennsylvania – require doctors to submit to the states' motor vehicle departments the names and addresses of people whom they have diagnosed as having or are treating for epilepsy. In these six states, both doctors and drivers who do not report the condition to the motor vehicle department may face civil or criminal liability if an accident occurs.

People with epilepsy may appeal the decision of a state department of motor vehicles to deny, fail to renew, or revoke a license. The appeal must be made within a specified period of time, determined by each state, following the agency's decision not to license.

Many states have adopted the federal medical qualifications for commercial licenses. People with epilepsy cannot be licensed to drive buses, including school buses, tractor trailers, and most trucks. They must meet the requirements for the operation of a passenger vehicle in order to be licensed to drive a taxi.

EMPLOYMENT

Under the employment provisions of the Americans with Disabilities Act (ADA) of 1990, a person with epilepsy cannot be denied a job unless he or she is actually unable to perform it. The person must have the education, skills, and experience required to hold a position and be able to accomplish the essential functions of the job with or without reasonable accommodation.

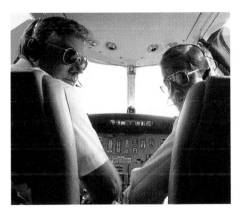

The significant terms are "essential functions" and "reasonable accommodation." The essential function requirement determines whether a person with epilepsy is qualified for a job. A function is essential if the job exists to perform it, only a limited number of employees can do it, or it is so specialized that a person is hired because of his or her expertise or ability to perform it. For example, driving is the essential function of bus

EXCLUDED PROFESSIONS
People with epilepsy cannot become airline pilots because a seizure while working would obviously put others in considerable danger.

and truck drivers, and people with epilepsy, who cannot obtain commercial driver's licenses, cannot perform those jobs. Driving is not, however, an essential function for a secretary who may be asked to run errands by car.

Reasonable accommodations are changes in the physical work area or in procedures that allow people with epilepsy to enjoy employment opportunities equal to those of people without epilepsy. It does not mean that jobs have to be adapted to meet the needs of applicants. Most people with epilepsy do not require such accommodations, which might include adjusting a computer display or installing a shield around machinery.

Applicants cannot be asked to disclose any condition they have, including epilepsy, either on an application form or at an interview. Medical examinations cannot be performed before a job is offered. Under federal, state, and local laws, however, some jobs require that applicants and employees have physical exams to determine their fitness to do a job. For example, airline pilots, bus and truck drivers, and construction workers must meet federal medical standards.

The Americans with Disabilities Act thus protects people with epilepsy from job discrimination based on stereotypes and myths about the condition. Each person's ability to do a job must be evaluated individually, which is important for those with epilepsy since the manifestation of seizures varies from person to person.

ASSESSING THE RISKS

One of the most important features of epilepsy is that it is an intermittent condition. If someone has poorly controlled epilepsy and has a seizure once a week, this still leaves 313 days in the year when the person is seizure-free.

It is thus important that a person does not let the epilepsy take over and control his or her life. Over-protection, excessive restrictions, and underachievement are far too common secondary handicaps of epilepsy, and they can be avoided. The main dangers of epilepsy come from its unpredictability, and certain precautions need to be taken.

It would be prudent to avoid certain high-risk activities, such as scuba diving, hang gliding, and mountain climbing, although well-organized mountain climbs are possible.

In most other circumstances, the social and psychological damage done by restricting a person's life probably outstrips the risks.

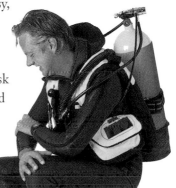

Swimming is possible but preferably should be done with someone who knows about the epilepsy and knows what to do should a seizure occur. The lifeguard or pool attendant should be informed. Bicycling and horse-back riding are also possible, but attention should be paid to the possible risks. Both of these pursuits need to be done with someone who knows about the epilepsy or in an organized group, and a helmet is mandatory.

ACTIVITIES TO AVOID
High-risk sports, such as scuba diving, should be avoided because seizures cannot be predicted.

At home, most activities carry only a small risk. However, certain precautions can be taken to minimize these risks. Showers are less risky than baths. If a bath is taken, the water should be shallow. Someone in the house should be informed, and the bathroom door should remain unlocked. A microwave is preferable to a stove, and pans containing hot oil should be avoided. Screens for open fires, radiators, and burners are advisable. In addition, alarms designed for people with epilepsy can be triggered if a person falls. They are useful for people with frequent seizures who live alone.

Frequent falls by someone with poorly controlled epilepsy can cause head and facial injuries. If these falls continue for long enough, a certain amount of brain damage and facial scarring can occur. In these people – very much a minority of people with epilepsy – wearing a protective helmet is advisable.

SCHOOLING AND PARENTING

It is wrong to generalize about a child with epilepsy. Epilepsy, as we hope is now apparent, describes many different conditions, has many different underlying causes, and occurs in many different people. It is inexcusable to label a person with epilepsy as an epileptic child or an epileptic adult and view such a person as a stereotype. Despite this, some important points about schooling have to be made.

GOING TO SCHOOL
Most children with epilepsy are able to attend mainstream schools.

Most children with epilepsy attend regular schools, and only the minority, who have both epilepsy and learning difficulties or very severe epilepsy, need special schools. (Advice about them is available from a number of organizations. See Useful addresses, pp.79–80.) Despite receiving mainstream education, many children with epilepsy underachieve at school for a variety of reasons. Both epilepsy itself and anticonvulsant drug treatment can impair a child's ability to learn. However, with modern drug management, there is less impairment of memory and greater control of seizures. A child with absence epilepsy can have many seizures that are unrecognized by both child and teacher, and instead appear to be lapses of concentration and poor class performance. Seizures at night can also affect a child's academic performance during the day.

More important, many children with epilepsy are almost expected by some to perform poorly, and this expectation by parents and teachers soon becomes self-fulfilling. Poor school attendance, low self-esteem, and anxieties about school are all likely to be major factors. There has to be good communication among school, parents, child, and doctor. It is important that school administrators know about the epilepsy and that teachers know what to do about seizures and understand the child's condition. Education packages for schools are available from a number of charitable organizations (see Useful addresses, pp.79–80).

In addition, it is important that neither teachers nor parents restrict the activities of a child unnecessarily (see Assessing the risks, pp.68–70). The child should be encouraged to think positively and to take part in school activities. Teachers should be aware of possible teasing and bullying. If it is likely that a child will have a seizure at school, it often is worth educating the class about seizures and epilepsy. It is important that the child does not feel or become isolated because of his or her seizures.

Overprotection by families, even of children with well-controlled epilepsy, is very common but counterproductive. This overprotection often persists into adulthood and can result in social isolation, poor social skills, dependency, childishness, underachievement, and low self-esteem. Striking a balance is understandably difficult, but it is important that this issue is not ignored. Parents should not be afraid to discuss their child's epilepsy with doctors, counselors, or others in order to gain a better understanding not only of their child's epilepsy but also of the restrictions that it will impose on their child's life. Many parents tend to err much too much on the side of overvigilance and overanxiety, and the potential for both psychological and social damage is great.

RELATIONSHIPS

In broad terms, people with epilepsy have fewer relationships and are often more isolated than normal. Prejudice among the general public is often blamed, but the actual causes of this are more complex. Some patients believe that there is a greater prejudice than actually exists. Together with parental overprotection, this can lead to fear of relationships. This anxiety often makes forming relationships more difficult, resulting in a certain amount of social isolation that only serves to fuel the original anxieties. Such concerns remain even when patients become seizure-free. Consequently, many people with epilepsy may need to be encouraged to think positively about themselves and their

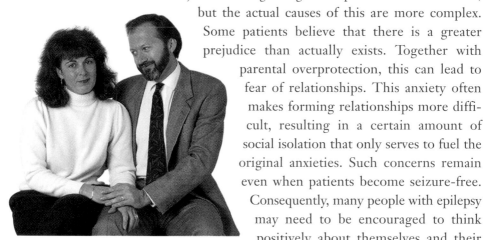

A TRUE PARTNERSHIP
There is no reason why someone with epilepsy should not enjoy a loving, fulfilling relationship. It may be difficult to tell a partner about your epilepsy, but it is important not to dwell on the negative aspects of the disease.

condition and to face their anxieties. Occasionally professional help is needed, and advice about this is available from a number of different sources (see Useful addresses, pp.79–80). It is important not to let epilepsy dominate one's life inappropriately because such a preoccupation can be self-destructive.

Once in a relationship, a person whose epilepsy is still active should inform his or her partner about it. There is no evidence to suggest that knowledge of a person's epilepsy is a major cause in the breakup of relationships. How and when to tell a partner can be difficult, but again the positive aspects of the condition should be emphasized, including the fact that epilepsy is usually easily controlled, is not inherited, and does not lead to mental illness. It is also possible for people with active epilepsy to have a family (see pp.62–64) and raise children. There is a danger of overdependency in some relationships and of treating the affected partner as a child, and both of these behaviors should be avoided.

PSYCHIATRIC DISEASE

The connection between psychiatric disease and seizures is complex. In the past, epilepsy was viewed as a form of psychiatric disease but now is considered a physical brain disease.

Psychiatric disease is, however, not uncommon in people with epilepsy. A person with epilepsy faces many social pressures and is more likely to be unemployed and single. It is therefore not surprising that anxiety and depression are common in those with epilepsy, especially those with a long history of poorly controlled seizures. However, both seizures and anticonvulsants can compound this depression through their effects on the brain and can occasionally themselves produce severe depression that may necessitate hospitalization and drug treatment.

Rarely, patients with temporal lobe epilepsy have episodes of paranoia and schizophrenia-like illnesses. These episodes are usually short-lived, occurring around the time of a seizure, just after a seizure, or between seizures. In a few individuals, these episodes may persist and may require long-term drug treatment. The exact association between temporal lobe epilepsy and psychosis is unclear, because both increases in seizure frequency (flurries of seizures) and decreases can result in psychotic episodes in some people.

Some psychiatric diseases and epilepsy have a common cause. For instance, severe brain damage at birth may lead to seizures, personality problems, and psychiatric disease. In these cases, it is not the epilepsy that causes the psychiatric problems but an underlying cause that results in both conditions.

KEY POINTS

- All people holding a driver's license must inform the state motor vehicle department if they have epileptic seizures.
- The Americans with Disabilities Act (ADA) of 1990 protects certain rights to employment.
- High-risk activities such as strenuous or dangerous sports should be avoided; most other sports can be enjoyed under some supervision.
- Parents of children with epilepsy should not be over-protective because this can result in their children's social isolation.
- Forming relationships can occasionally be difficult for people with epilepsy, but people with epilepsy must be careful not to let the condition control their lives.

Overall outlook

With appropriate care and treatment, most people with epilepsy can look forward to a normal and fulfilling life with a normal life expectancy.

THE LIKELY OUTCOME

The outlook or prognosis of a condition is the "forecast" for that condition; it tells us what is likely to happen in the future. As was explained in the introduction, epilepsy clears up in most people and, therefore, it has a good prognosis. About 80 percent of people who take anticonvulsant medication become seizure-free, after which the decision about if and when to stop the medication arises. It is usual to wait for a patient to be seizure-free for about two years before stopping medication. There are a number of factors that determine the chances of success or failure in withdrawing drugs, including the underlying cause of the epilepsy. Overall, however, about 60 percent of patients who have been seizure-free for two years successfully stop taking drugs.

The chances of discontinuing the medication are better in the young and in those taking only one anticonvulsant. However, some people do not wish to risk

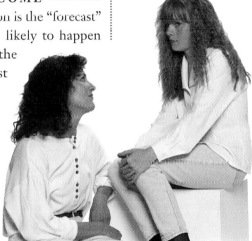

A POSITIVE OUTLOOK
Young people are more likely to remain seizure-free than are adults when medication is stopped.

not taking their drugs, because the social consequences of having a seizure may be too great.

These social consequences tend to be greater in adults than in children. Indeed, because of the better chances of withdrawing medication, the lesser consequences of having a seizure, and the potentially negative effects of medication on schooling, seizure-free children are often the group that benefit most from discontinuing anticonvulsants.

One of the questions that has been the subject of debate for many years is whether anticonvulsants themselves help cure the condition as well as stop seizures. The answer to this question is unknown. Recently, however, studies have demonstrated that even late anticonvulsant treatment probably carries the same good prognosis as early drug treatment.

MENTAL AND PHYSICAL HEALTH

There is often concern that epilepsy and seizures will commonly lead to mental and physical deterioration. This is not so. In most people, seizures stop or are well controlled by anticonvulsants, and these individuals usually lead normal lives. Unfortunately, a few people who suffer uncontrolled seizures may also experience mental and physical deterioration. In these cases, however, the deterioration is usually due to the underlying cause of the epilepsy or injuries that occur during the seizures, not the seizures themselves.

The possible development of mental illness is often another concern. However, as has already been explained, mental illness directly attributable to seizures is rare, and seizures themselves rarely lead to the destruction of personality and mind.

DEATH AND EPILEPSY

Does epilepsy affect life expectancy? The answer is that poorly controlled, severe epilepsy most certainly does, and even people with well-controlled epilepsy may have a slightly shortened life expectancy. The reasons for this are not altogether certain, but in a number of cases the underlying cause of the epilepsy (e.g., a brain tumor) may shorten life expectancy. In addition, people with epilepsy are at a higher risk of accidents, which usually occur while having a seizure or as the result of the seizure. Sudden unexpected death, a sudden, unwitnessed death of a previously healthy person for which no cause is found, is more common in those with epilepsy and may be as high as one in 400 people with epilepsy per year, and probably higher in people with severe epilepsy. The reasons for this are also unclear, but it may be the result of an unwitnessed seizure.

Having said this, most seizures do not result in death or brain damage. It is certain, however, that people with well-controlled epilepsy do better than those with poorly controlled epilepsy. As treatment continues to improve, the prognosis for epilepsy, the lives, and even the life expectancy of those with epilepsy will improve along with it.

KEY POINTS

- Epilepsy clears up in most people.
- People with epilepsy can reduce or prevent their seizures with drugs and can then lead normal lives.
- Seizures rarely cause brain damage or death.

Summary

In this book, there are a number of important points that deserve emphasis.

- Epilepsy is a common and treatable condition.
- A seizure results from an "electrical storm" in the brain, and the form of a seizure depends on where it starts and how far it spreads.
- A number of conditions can be confused with seizures.
- There are a multitude of causes of seizures.
- Febrile convulsions rarely lead to epilepsy.
- Most cases of people with epilepsy are well controlled with drugs, which must be taken regularly.
- Doses of anticonvulsant drugs are determined by balancing seizure control against drug side effects.
- Anticonvulsant blood levels are merely a guide to drug doses.
- Epilepsy gets better and clears up in many people.
- The prognosis for people with epilepsy probably relates to the underlying cause.
- Brain surgery is successful in and suitable for a number of patients with drug-resistant epilepsy.
- Most prejudice against people with epilepsy is unjust, but it is often not as great as the person with epilepsy believes.
- Most people with epilepsy can lead normal lives and should not be over-protected.
- Finally, the word *epileptic* is an adjective that should be confined to the phrase "epileptic seizure" and should not be used either to describe or to stereotype people.

Useful addresses

ASSESSMENT CENTERS FOR EPILEPSY

In the US, there are a number of specialized assessment centers for epilepsy, some of which may specialize in either adults or children. In addition to these, there are specialized units in many regional neurological centers. These units specialize in the assessment of patients with epilepsy, especially those patients who are resistant to anticonvulsant treatment.

SPECIAL SCHOOLS FOR CHILDREN WITH EPILEPSY

Most children with epilepsy receive mainstream schooling. There are, however, children with severe epilepsy who have learning difficulties or behavioral problems that preclude them from mainstream education.

These children are often eligible for residential schooling in a specialized center where there is medical supervision.

Although there are no special schools for children with epilepsy in the US, try calling the Department for Special Education Services of your local board of education for names of schools that offer the appropriate supervision for your child.

There are also certain national organizations that can help, including the National Department of Disabilities and Special Needs (1-888-DSN-INFO) and the National Information Center for Handicapped Children and Youth (1-800-999-5599).

Various parent advocacy groups have networks for families of children with epilepsy. Try the Department of Children and Youth with Epilepsy within the Epilepsy Foundation of America, (301) 459-3700, and Parent Advocacy Coalition for Education Rights (PACER), (800) 53-PACER.

EPILEPSY ORGANIZATIONS

There are a number of charitable organizations providing information about epilepsy, educating the general public about epilepsy, organizing meetings, and funding research. Some of these organizations run information services and provide videos and information packages for schools. The Epilepsy Foundation of America is the main association in the US and has a local community network.

American Academy of Neurology
Online: www.aan.com
2221 University Avenue SW, Suite 335
Minneapolis, MN 55414
Tel: (612) 623-8115

American Epilepsy Society
Online: www.aesnet.org
638 Prospect Avenue
Hartford, CT 06105-4240
Tel: (860) 586-7505
Fax: (860) 586-7550

The Comprehensive Epilepsy Center
Columbia-Presbyterian Medical Center
Neurological Institute
710 West 168th Street
New York, NY 10032
Tel: (212) 305-1742
Fax: (212) 305-1450

Epilepsy Foundation of America
Online: www.efa.com
4351 Garden City Drive
Landover, MD 20785
Tel: (800) EFA-1000
Tel: (301) 459-3700
Fax: (301) 577-4941

Epilepsy Information Service
Tel: (800) 642-0500

Epilepsy International
Online: www.epiworld.com

Massachusetts General Hospital
Epilepsy Unit at Harvard Medical School
Online: www.neurosurgery.mgh.harvard.edu
55 Fruit Street
Boston, MA 02114
Tel: (617) 726-3311
Fax: (617) 726-7546

University of Pennsylvania Epilepsy
Center
Online: www.med.upenn.edu
University of Pennsylvania Medical Center
Department of Neurology
3 West Gates
3400 Spruce Street
Philadelphia, PA 19104
Tel: (215) 349-5166

Texas Neurosciences Institute
Comprehensive Epilepsy Center
Online: www.texasneurosciences.com
4410 Medical Drive
Suite 660
San Antonio, TX 78229
Tel: (210) 615-8070
Fax: (210) 615-6645

Washington University Epilepsy Program
660 South Euclid Street
St. Louis, MO 63110
Tel: (314) 362-3888
Fax: (314) 362-0296

Glossary

Adherence: taking a drug and following medical advice as instructed.

Aura: the warning that may occur before a major seizure or in isolation; a simple partial seizure.

Computerized tomography (CT): a brain scan using X rays and computer analysis to form detailed pictures of slices through the brain.

Dysplasia: the abnormal development of cells in the brain.

Electroencephalography (EEG): the recording of brain waves (the electrical activity within the brain).

Epileptic seizures: the result of an electrical storm in the brain. They are divided into partial seizures (simple partial, complex partial, and secondary generalized), which begin in one part of the brain but can spread to other parts, and generalized seizures (tonic-clonic, clonic, tonic, absence seizures, and myoclonus), which begin in both hemispheres of the brain at once.

Febrile convulsions: seizures that occur in children with fever, only rarely leading to epilepsy.

Hemispheres: the two halves of the brain. In most people, the left hemisphere is "dominant" and controls language.

Hippocampus: a part of the temporal lobe (see **Lobes**) involved in the formation of memories. Damage to this area commonly causes epilepsy.

Hyperventilation: overbreathing, which can occasionally be confused with an epileptic seizure.

Idiosyncratic side effects: side effects that occur only in certain people. The most common such side effect of anticonvulsant drugs is rash.

Lobes: different parts of the brain determined by position, each of which has a particular set of functions. The frontal lobe is at the front and deals with movement, the parietal lobe is in the middle and deals with sensation, the occipital lobe is at the back and deals with sight, and the temporal lobe is at the side and deals with memory formation.

Magnetic resonance imaging (MRI): the use of a strong magnetic field and radio waves to cause the vibration of atoms that give off energy, which is then turned into a detailed picture of the brain by computer analysis. MRI is a more effective test than CT scanning in detecting brain abnormalities that cause epilepsy.

Monotherapy: treatment with one drug.

Pharmacoresistant epilepsy: resistance to anticonvulsant therapy in a minority of people with epilepsy. It is also known as refractory or drug-resistant epilepsy.

Photosensitivity: propensity to seizures after exposure to flashing lights; present in about one in 20 people with epilepsy.

Polytherapy: treatment with two or more drugs.

Prognosis: the "forecast" or estimate of outcome for a condition.

Pseudoseizures: seizures that are not epileptic but are like an emotional outburst and usually due to deep-rooted psychological problems. They

do not respond to anticonvulsant treatment and can be difficult to distinguish from epileptic seizures.

Sodium amytal test: an injection of the anesthetic sodium amytal into the blood supply to each half of the brain in turn to determine the possible effects of epilepsy surgery on memory and language.

Status epilepticus: a seizure, or series of seizures, in which consciousness is lost for over 30 minutes. Prolonged convulsion (convulsive status epilepticus) is a medical emergency, and the patient should be taken to the hospital immediately.

Syncope: a faint or a sudden loss of consciousness.

Video telemetry: simultaneous recording of EEG with video, used to monitor patients who are difficult to diagnose and for assessment before epilepsy surgery.

Notes

Notes

Index

P

panic attacks 24
paranoia 73
parenting implications 70–73
parietal lobe, overview 11–13
partial seizures
  causes 16–17
  drug treatments 40, 51–3, 56
  migraine confusion 23–4
  overview 12–15
  syncope confusion 23
Paul, St. 7
"petit mal" attacks see absence seizures
pharmacoresistant patients 47
phenobarbital 37, 40, 52
  breast feeding 64
phenytoin 40, 53
photosensitivity, triggers 36–7
polytherapy 43, 63
postictal phase 15
potassium bromide 8, 37
pregnancy 58, 62–4
primary generalized epilepsy 20–1, 35
primidone 40, 54
protective helmets 69–70
"pseudoseizures" 24–5
psychiatric assessments 49
psychiatric disease 73–4, 76
psychological testing 48

R

record-keeping 45
recovery, statistics 9, 19, 75
recovery position 33
reflex epilepsies 34
reflexes, testing 26
refractory patients 47
relationship implications 72–3
relaxation benefits 35
risk assessment 68–9, 77

S

schizophrenia 73
schooling implications 70–71
secondary generalized seizures 14–15
seizures 18–19, 23–7
  see also convulsions
  classification 12–13
  driving implications 65–7
  drug treatments list 40
  first aid treatment 32–3, 59–60
  longer term treatment 34–50
  overview 10–21
  psychiatric disease 73–4, 76
  record keeping 45
  sports 69
  types 12–16, 61–2
side effects, drug treatments 39–43, 51–8, 62–4
simple partial seizures
  diagnosis 23
  overview 12–13
sleep deprivation, triggers 35
smell 10
social implications 65–74, 76
sodium amytal test 49
spikes, EEGs 27
spina bifida 63
sports 69–7
statistics 8–9, 18, 46
  surgery results 50
status epilepticus 61–2
stress, triggers 35
summary 78
sunglasses, benefits 36
suppositories, diazepam usage 33–4, 58, 60–61
surgery
  criteria 47
  overview 46–50
  preliminary tests 48–9
  results 49–50

sweet sensations 10
symptom concept 19, 29
syncope 22–3
syndromes, concept 19–21

T

television, triggers 36–7
temporal lobe
  overview 11–13
  psychiatric disease 73–4
tiagabine hydrochloride 56
tolerance, drug treatments 52, 56
tonic seizures 14–15
tonic-clonic seizures 14–15, 51, 53
topiramate 40, 56
treatment
  see also individual drugs; surgery
  first aid 32–3, 59–60
  longer-term 34–50
  overview 32–50
  seizures 32–4, 59–62
  trigger avoidance 34–7
triggers 34–7, 11, 59–60
  see also causes

U

useful addresses 79–80

V

valproate sodium 40, 53–4
video telemetry 27
vision disturbances 23–4
vitamin depletion, drug-treatment-related 53–4, 57, 63–4

W

weight gains 53
West syndrome 19

X

X-rays, CT scanning 28

Acknowledgments

PUBLISHER'S ACKNOWLEDGMENTS
Dorling Kindersley Publishing, Inc. would like to thank the following for their help and participation in this project:

Managing Editor Stephanie Jackson; **Managing Art Editor** Nigel Duffield;
Editorial Assistance Janel Bragg, Mary Lindsay, Jennifer Quasha, Ashley Ren, Design Revolution;
Design Assistance Sarah Hall, Marianne Markham, Design Revolution, Chris Walker; **Production** Michelle Thomas, Elizabeth Cherry.

Consultancy Dr. Tony Smith, Dr. Sue Davidson;
Indexing Indexing Specialists, Hove; **Administration** Christopher Gordon.

Illustrations (p.60) ©Philip Wilson.

Picture Research Angela Anderson, Andy Sansom;
Picture Librarian Charlotte Oster.

PICTURE CREDITS
The publisher would like to thank the following for their kind permission to reproduce their photographs. Every effort has been made to trace the copyright holders. Dorling Kindersley Publishing apologizes for any unintentional omissions and would be pleased, in any such cases, to add an acknowledgment in future editions.

APM p.45; **Corbis** p.50 (R. W. Jones); **Musée d'Orsay** p.7 (Philippe Sebert);
Pictor Uniphoto p.67; **Science Photo Library** p.12 (Keith Hunt),
p.14 (BSIP VEM), p.28 (BSIP ESTIOT), p.3, p.29 (Meham Kulyk);
Telegraph Colour Library p.47 (H. Sykes).